Princess Priscilla's
Quest for the Zany Zombies

By Philip L. Levin, MD

For Lex:

Chase Those Zombies!

Philip Levin

11/5/16

Princess Priscilla's Quest for the Zany Zombies

By Philip L. Levin, MD

Illustrations by Saga

Philip L. Levin
PO Box 4808
Biloxi, MS 39535
writerpllevin@gmail.com

Text by Philip L. Levin, MD
Illustrations by Saga
©2016 Doctor's Dreams Publishing
All Rights Reserved

Published by
Doctor's Dreams Publishing
P O Box 4808
Biloxi, MS 39535, USA

Prepared in the United States of America
Printed in Korea by Pacom Press

ISBN: 978-1-942181-08-8
LOC: 2016911242

Chapter One:
The Drought

Princess Priscilla leaned out of her castle window and waved the short wand in little circles. With eyes closed she shouted, "Rain, Bane, for Puddlin' Shame!" Stepping back, she turned in circles three times and threw the stick as far as she could out the window. "You see any rain?"

Priscilla turned to her pet troll, cute as could be in his miniature suit, tailored to his green-skinned half-human / half-frog figure. Rashpewkin jumped up on the windowsill next to her and held his three-fingered hand over his brow to shade his eyes. "Nope a-roonie."

Brushing back her long blond tresses, Priscilla wiped her forehead with her handkerchief. "I should have known a wand that only cost a single gold coin wouldn't work. That peddler cheated us."

"Rip-a-dee-doo off," Rashpewkin said in agreement. Pointing down at the half-dried up moat he sighed. "No rain in Kingdom two moons. See moat monster tail."

Priscilla looked at where he pointed and just caught a glimpse of a three prong pointed tail splashing back under the water.

"Rashpewkin hungry," the little troll said. He rubbed his hand against his stomach, casting her a droopy-eyed look.

"Me too. Come on, let's head down to the castle keep and see if Coretta found anything to cook." She led her pet down the twisting tower stairs into the kitchen where the cook, Coretta, was stirring a gray bubbling porridge in a back iron pot.

Coretta dipped in a ladle and plopped a dollop of the slop into a bowl held by a curly-haired girl perched on a pink polka-dot toadstool. The child, about four years old, wore a red-checkered vest, a short red skirt, red shoes, and red ribbons hanging on each of a half dozen strands of dark curls.

Dipping her spoon into her bowl, the girl brought out a small smidgen of the white sizzling mixture and, following a sniff, gave a pouty grimace.

"Yuck." Looking over at Coretta, she asked, "Is this all we got?"

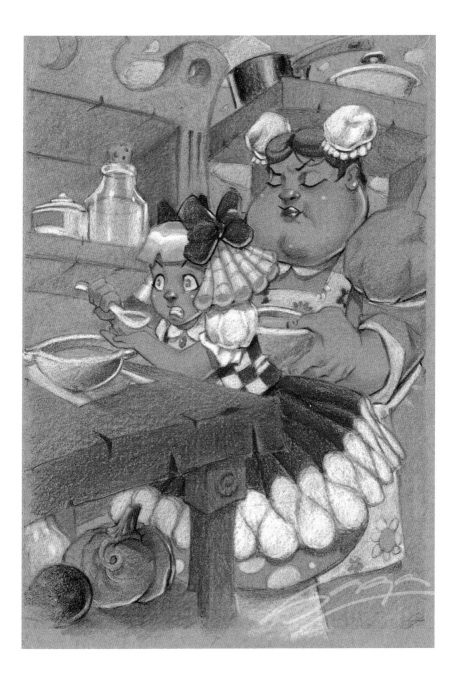

Coretta dipped her ladle into a second pot and dumped a dark gray clump on top.

"You say you're hungry, so don't be grumpy. For curds you say, now eat your whey."

"Which way?" the girl asked.

Priscilla peeked into the girl's bowl, stepping away at the sight of the ugly mixture. "Who are you?" she asked the urchin.

The child hopped off the stool and curtsied. "I be Mary, if it please Your Highness." She sat back on the stool and touched the spoon into the bowl, bringing up a morsel of grey gunk for a lick. Her eyes opened wide. "Hey, this be good!" Pushing her spoon deeper into the bowl, she brought up a small mountain of the sticky white and grey mash, smearing as much on her face as getting into her mouth. Priscilla picked up a wet cloth and dabbed at the girl's face.

"Where did you come from?" the princess asked.

"Me family's come down from over Rhyme Town," the child answered.

Coretta spoke up, "Mary be my niece, if you leave her in peace. Rhyme Town is my home, the place of the poem. There creek is all dry, no rain in the sky. They having swift feet, they're coming for eats."

"Dragon's dirt! More mouths to feed! Well, we certainly can't let the peasants starve."

As the girl ate, a big spider floated down on a shining silk string, hovering just above her head. Rashpewkin leaped a somersault over her head, capturing the arachnid with his long tongue on the way. Mary barely glanced at him before going back to her food.

Rashpewkin crawled around the floor looking for bugs to eat, not following Priscilla who accompanied the girl as she carried her half-finished bowl into the next room where they found four boys of about five years old. The first, with long overalls and choppy blonde hair, sat on a rickety tall stool in a corner.

"Hi Jack," Mary called, and he leaned down to kiss her cheek. He doffed his cap at Priscilla.

"Your Highness." Turning to Mary, he said, "You're not your usual contrary self this morning. What's up, Sis?"

She held up the bowl. "A bit of curds and whey. You hungry?"

The boy stuck in his thumb, but it came out bare. "No plums?" He leaned back on the stool and closed his eyes.

Across the room one of the other boys hopped back and forth over a burning candle while the other two cheered him on.

"Forty-three," said the one jumping, his green tunic and rope-tied pants rippling as he moved. Bright red hair topped his face full of freckles. His feet barely touched the floor before he bent his

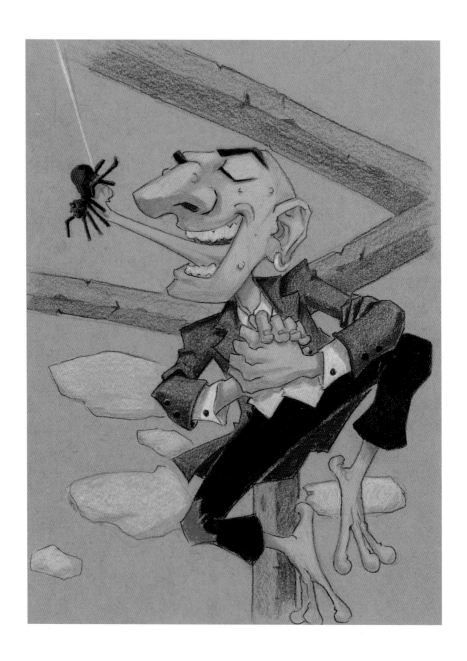

legs and hopped back across the flame.

"Forty-four," announced one of the other boys, wearing an oversized shirt. He held a little harp that seemed to be playing all by itself.

When the candle jumper spotted the princess, he stopped jumping and gave a deep bow. The other boys, seeing their brother's action, followed suit. "Your Highness," they all said.

Mary pointed to the three. "This be my nimble brother Jack," indicating the candle jumper, "and this be my climbing brother Jack," pointing at the third boy. Turning to the fourth boy, a very thin child wearing scraps of pants with patches on both knees, she said, "This be my hungry brother Jack."

Priscilla curtsied in response to their bows. "Your mother couldn't think of any names besides Jack?" she asked.

Mary handed over the bowl to the candle jumper, who took two spoonfuls. "No fat," he said, "so you can eat this, Jack." He handed it to the boy in scraps. This one proceeded to lick the bowl vigorously.

"Does he always do that?" Priscilla asked. "He eats just like my troll."

The thin boy handed the bowl back to his sister who showed it to Priscilla. "See? Licked clean."

"Yep, just like my troll."

"Why are they all named Jack?" Priscilla asked.

"Daddy loved Jack stuff," one of the Jacks explained. "He played blackjack with his friends, and his favorite poker game was 'All Jacks Wild.'"

"Which he used to call out when he came home," another Jack said. "He'd fish for amberjacks, eat applejacks, wore bootjacks, worked as a crackerjack lumberjack, unless he was on the road, when he'd highjack a carjack."

"We had pets at home," the third Jack added. "Jackrabbits, jackals and jackdaws. We ate jackfish and wore matching jackets."

"He came to no good, though," the fourth Jack said sadly. "Drank so much jackfruit juice he got jackhammered and ended up in a straightjacket."

"What was your Daddy's name?" Princess Priscilla asked.

"Peter Peter," Mary said. "He used to love eating Jack-o-lanterns." She sighed. "That 'twas when we had pumpkins. Now e'reything's so dry, we ain't got nothing." She looked up at the princess. "You gotta DO something, Princess. We gotta have rain."

The four boys joined in. "Yes, please Your Highness. The whole Kingdom needs your help or we'll all starve."

Priscilla patted each on the head. "I certainly will."

Giving the girl a hug, the princess went back to the kitchen. There she found Rashpewkin sitting across the table from Coretta playing a game. Each player moved small pieces around a checkered pattern made on the table. Priscilla settled next to them.

Rashpewkin slid a carved horseman into one of Coretta's peasants, knocking it down. She stared in surprise. "I hate to say this is my fate, but now I find I'm in checkmate."

"Game's over?" Priscilla asked. Receiving their nods, she said, "Then let's talk turkey - well not just turkey, but about any food. Our cupboards are bare, the garden's not producing, and trade has dried up. Now we have another five mouths to feed. What are we going to do about this drought?"

The troll lifted his foot to scratch behind his ear. "Deeper well? Rashpewkin like digging holes. Find worms to eat."

Priscilla shook her head. "It'd take too long and might not reach water. Why isn't it raining?"

Coretta shushed them with a finger to her mouth and looked stealthily around the room. She whispered, "It's Magic here, I can swear. For drought to burst, must beat the curse."

"Curse?" Rashpewkin dropped to the floor, curled into a ball, and rolled himself into a cupboard, shutting the door behind him.

Priscilla grasped Coretta's hands. "Curse? What curse? How

are we going to break it?"

Coretta pulled back her hands, stood and turned to the fireplace where she stirred a slowly-bubbling brew. "I'm sure I'll be the last to shout, how to snuff a curse on out. You leave me free, you buzzing bee. Take your troll on down the road, visit the men who deal in grim."

Priscilla stood and nodded. "Okay, I get it." She opened up the cabinet door and pulled her pet out by his arm. "Come on, Pewker. We've got a visit to make in the village."

She pulled on her bonnet and grabbed her purse.

Taking her hand, he asked, "A visit? Who we visit?"

"We need to find a bit of magic to break this curse." They crossed the drawbridge and headed down the cobblestone path towards the village.

Just before they passed around the bend, Coretta called out to them, "Be you so kind, if you wouldn't mind, if you're in the right mood, bring back some food!"

Chapter Two:
At the Fair

Princess Priscilla always loved the walk down to the village, a trip she took every week or so. The castle, being a bit isolated at the top of a hill, surrounded by a moat, and near the edge of the Mystic Forest, did not receive a lot of visitors. Coming down to the village provided a pleasant change of scenery with opportunities for entertainment.

Priscilla and Rashpewkin strolled at a leisurely pace, often stopping to talk with the farmers they'd meet on the road or in nearby fields, or just to look at interesting flowers or animals they'd pass. About an hour into the walk they came upon a large white rabbit perched on an overturned log just off the path. The bunny pulled a pocket watch out of his waistcoat and muttered something about being very late before hopping away into the bushes.

Princess Priscilla grabbed Rashpewkin to prevent him from chasing it. "Let it be," she ordered.

He cocked his head to look up at her. "Make rabbit stew? Princess miss lunch. Be hungry."

She put a hand on her tummy, feeling it rumble at the suggestion. "We can pick up something in town. We're not out camping, you know."

"No matter me." He popped out his long tongue and snagged a cocoon off a branch, chewing a bit before spitting out a green splat. "Not ripe."

"Yuck. You sure have a lot of frog in you. I thought you'd be more boyish when you turned."

Rashpewkin shrugged and hopped over to a nest of spiders where he began picking them out and popping them into his mouth.

Priscilla rested on the log the bunny had been on. She watched a fox leap several times trying to reach some grapes. After several failed attempts he turned his back on them, tail high in the air, and strolled off. *Probably sour anyway,* Priscilla thought.

With the dry air, the sun seemed extra hot, and the princess felt sweat bead on her forehead. She took a drink from the water skin they'd brought before standing to resume her walk. "I hope we can find someone magical in the village who knows how to break the curse. Let's keep our eyes open for a magician or sorcerer or such."

Rashpewkin turned a nervous eye in her direction. "Not evil one?"

The princess shrugged. "We'll see who we can find."

Walking into the main square of the village, they found a shindig in progress. Jugglers, bards, and acrobats gathered onlookers who applauded their antics, rewarding good performances with a few coins in set-up hats. Along the park edges, vendors had tables laden with foods, weavings, and a wide variety of knickknacks.

A young man dressed in a blue military uniform bowed deeply to them. The princess liked his looks; his sandy hair lay in bangs across his forehead above sharp blue eyes that glittered with good humor. In one arm he cuddled a twisted brass horn, its shape reminding Priscilla of the bugle the Royal Horn Blower used to blow at the king's functions, before the blower got too old to blow. "Welcome, Royal Highness," the man in blue said.

"Welcome yourself," she replied. "Who are you and what do you do?"

"They called me Little Boy Blue when I was in the royal army where I blew boogie woogie for Company B. At the moment I'm in between jobs. Perhaps you need a horn-blower in the castle?"

Rashpewkin hopped over and ran his finger along the edge of the horn. "Shiny!" he said.

"How good are you at blowing your horn?" the princess asked.

"I'm so good, I can control any mammal. When I was a shepherd boy, I kept the sheep in the meadow and the cows out of the corn. Last month I played such a catchy tune, I rid an entire town of its rats!" He brought his instrument to his lips and let out such a lively jig that the princess found herself tapping one foot, and then the other. Looking over at Rashpewkin, she saw him dancing in circles, snapping his fingers in joy.

"Stop, stop," she cried. "I'm convinced."

Boy Blue put down his horn and smiled. "Job at the castle?"

"Maybe." The princess patted down her hair, replacing a curl or two loosened by her dancing. "Meanwhile, tell us what's going on here today."

"It's the festival of the fall harvest moon when everyone from miles around comes to the fair. There's everything you could want here today, from pumpkins to peppermint."

"Well good, 'cause I'm hungry. Let's see if we can find something to eat."

The three strolled around the square and Priscilla paused

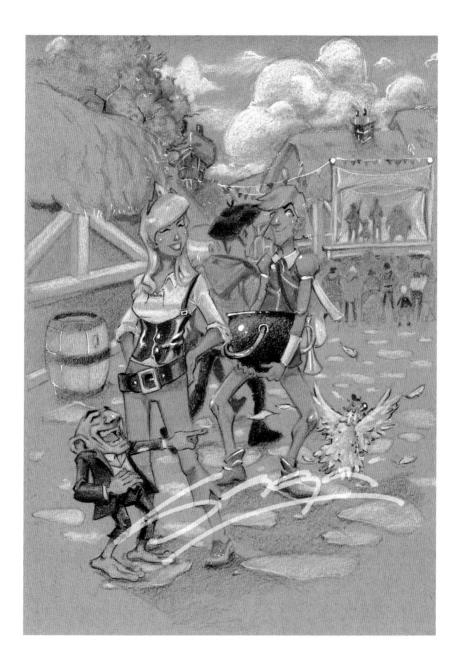

to look at a table holding four pies. The banner draped across the display's front claimed each pie contained two-dozen blackbirds. That didn't seem very appetizing, and she hurried on.

Another table held three pots. Priscilla asked the vendor what was in each.

"They all hold pease porridge," the seller replied. "This one is scalding hot, and this one is so cold it's formed a solid block."

"What about the third one?"

"This is last week's porridge. It's nine days old."

The princess decided none of them appealed to her and moved on.

The next booth held a sign reading, "Goldilocks's 'just right' stew." In the middle of the otherwise empty table stood a small pot. Behind the table sat a chubby little girl dressed in lederhosen, her blonde hair braided into two long cords on the sides of her head. She knocked the side of the old gray pot with her ladle and offered them stew.

Priscilla peered into the pot and saw it empty. "How are you going to feed us from an empty pot?"

"It's a magic pot, given to me by my Uncle Grimm."

"Why he so grim?" Rashpewkin asked.

"That was his name," she explained. "It was my other uncle's name too. They were two too-grim Grimms. You hungry, Your Highness? I can feed all three of you for one leprechaun dugget."

The princess pulled the coin out of her purse and held it up. "Let me see the food first."

The girl leaned over the pot and said, "Cook, little pot, cook." A delicious aroma came up from the old receptacle as it began to fill itself with thick vegetable stew. Once it was full, "Stop, little pot, stop," she said. She ladled out three bowls of the meaty broth and the princess handed her the coin.

"That sure would be nice to have back at the castle," Priscilla told her. "Is it for sale?"

The girl, who was busy spooning the remainders into her mouth, shook her head. "It was given to my uncle by his son, the boy who climbed to the top of the beanstalk." Looking up, she asked, "Do you know Jack?"

"I think I met him this morning. In fact, I think maybe he's at the castle now with his other brothers Jack and sister Mary. They're all very hungry."

Goldilocks scratched her chin as she considered. "Well … I suppose I could rent it to you for a few days—say at two duggets a day?"

"I'll take it for four days." The princess took another eight duggets from her coin pouch and handed them over. She gave the magic pot to Boy Blue to carry for her.

Priscilla, Rashpewkin, and Boy Blue walked out to the center of the square, eating their stew. Feeling a pecking at her trousers, Priscilla looked down to find a little chicken trying to eat a loose thread from the princess's pantaloons. Priscilla took a spoonful of her stew and dropped it onto the bird's head. The bird ran off shouting, "The sky is falling! The sky is falling!"

In the middle of the village square stood a large stage with a big sign overhead proclaiming, "Welcome to the Bare Bear Fair Fare Fair." She asked Boy Blue to explain the event.

He indicated the stage where three men wearing only bear hats and hairy pants stood preening. "It's a beauty contest, see? Contestants get to pay a fare to climb on stage and pick which of the bare bears is the fairest."

As they watched, Goldilocks climbed up on stage. She walked along the line slowly, stopping by each to look him up and down. Shaking her head at the first one, she said, "Too skinny." To the second, "Too big." She circled the third one twice before announcing, "He's just right."

The crowd applauded, and, after paying her fare from the duggets she'd just received, she and her bear went off stage together.

The princess scanned the tents along the edge of the square. "Look!" she said, pointing across the yard. "There's a magical fairy tent over there. Let's go see."

"Those things make me nervous," Boy Blue said. "I'll meet up with you when you're done."

Chapter Three:
Freda the Fair

The princess and Rashpewkin made their way through the crowd to the little tent, its purple drapes slung over a frame of golden poles, each topped with a tiny statue of a mythical being. Gold embroidered runes hung on the entrance and at each corner. Pulling the flap open, Priscilla stepped inside. Rashpewkin peeked in through the tent flaps.

The space stretched out in all directions for what seemed like forever, fading into darkness. About a dozen yards into the room a round glass tabletop hovered in the air with a milky glass sphere on its surface.

As Priscilla approached the table, a chair materialized on her side and a wavering feminine voice spoke. "Please sit down, young lady."

The princess stood behind the chair, holding onto its back and squinting into the darkness in all directions. Besides a bit of illumination from the tent flap behind her, the only other light came from the glass ball. It washed over Priscilla like a warm bath, soothing and tingling. She settled onto the chair, which moved her up to the table. The globe before her began to swirl in a kaleidoscope of colors, showing brief, somewhat familiar images, before scrambling again.

The princess startled when she looked up and found an old woman sitting on the other side of the table. Silver hair, mostly tied up into a bun, leaked out in a splay around her head like a pincushion. Sapphire eyes peered out under a brow creased with friendly lines. Below a long hooked nose decorated with a two-hair mole, thin white lips pressed together, turning up at each corner in a bewitching smile.

"Why, hello," Priscilla managed to say through her surprise. "You must be … um …"

"Freda the Fair Fairy at your service." The sorceress waved her hands and a dozen glowing butterflies fluttered out of them and into the darkness.

"You frightened me," Priscilla said. "Why did you appear so suddenly?"

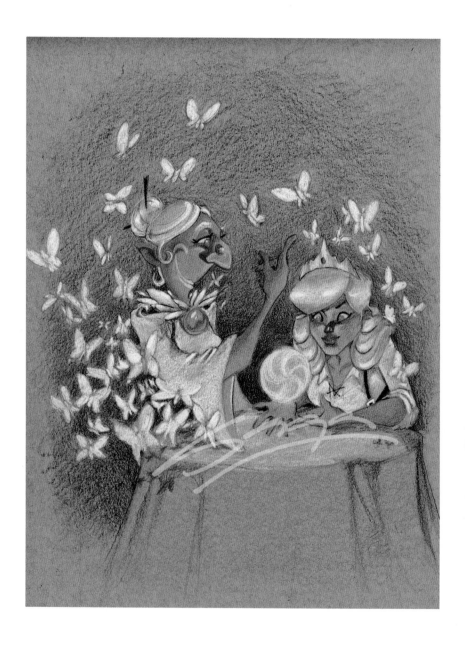

"I always stay hidden until I'm sure its safe. You'd be surprised how many people want to strike a happy medium." She pointed at Rashpewkin who still cowered at the tent flap. "And who is that strange creature lurking at the doorway? Come closer you little troll – let me have a look at you."

Rashpewkin hopped up and crouched behind Priscilla, hiding his head between his legs and tucking his hands on top.

The sorceress made a sweeping motion with her hand, and the chair holding the princess rotated a quarter way around the table leaving the troll exposed. The globe brightened, casting a white beam onto the green creature.

"Look at me," Freda commanded.

He unwound, cocking up his head and giving a feeble smile. "Howdy-doo."

"So, it is you, Rashpewkin." She looked him over and broke into a silly giggle. "I don't think I've ever seen such a creature. You're half-man / half-frog, aren't you? You look ridiculous."

Rashpewkin shrugged, his green limbs swinging like an undulating tent. He hopped back and forth, sticking out his long tongue and licking his ear with it. With a couple of hops he landed beside Priscilla, who climbed off her chair and gave him a hug.

"Don't be mean!" the princess scolded. "He's a sweet creature."

Freda looked down at Rashpewkin who hid his face against Priscilla's back. "I don't suppose he ever told you how he got into this fix in the first place?" the fairy asked.

The princess shook her head.

"I was out with my friend, He-Man, in the Royal Kingdom of Eternia, where I'd set up my tent at the Festival of the Two-Horned Unicorns. All sorts of clients came visiting: a serpent woman with forked tongue, a carpenter with a hammertoe, and an invisible spy who'd been spotted. It was in dispelling this last client that your friend here got into trouble. He and his cousin had snuck under the back edge of my tent. When I cast the despotting spell on the spy, the ward wandered off the worm and floated down on the two young royals. Naturally, it turned them both into frogs. You should have heard them croak. Well, I don't mean they died – just sang in coarse chorus."

She turned back to Rashpewkin. "So how'd you become this troll? Oh, wait a minute. I bet I know." Turning to Priscilla she said, "You didn't? Oh, you DID! You KISSED him, didn't you?"

The princess eyebrows tightened in a scowl. "Normally I don't go for slimy things. But there was Rashpewkin, looking so cute on a big lily pad and croaking a song. I mean, he obviously wasn't your normal frog, being almost two feet tall. My mother used to tell me that kissing an enchanted frog would turn him into a prince." She leaned forward, holding her palm cupped against her face, so only Freda could hear her next words. "He actually wasn't the first frog I kissed, though the only one who the kiss ever changed."

Freda sat back and waved her hand over the globe. It created a swirl of colors before coalescing into the profile of a woman. Priscilla gasped, recognizing her Auntie Em.

"Yes," the fairy said. "I knew your auntie well. Did you know she bought the love potion she gave your uncle from me? Ah, that was a wedding for the ages, yes indeed. For the ages." She sat back and sighed, her eyes closed.

Priscilla waited patiently until she heard the woman snore. The princess reached her foot under the table and gave the fairy's shin a little kick.

Freda's eyes popped open. "Where were we?"

"I was telling you about when I kissed Rashpewkin and he turned from an overgrown frog into a half-frog/half-boy. How come he didn't turn into a handsome prince?"

Freda rubbed her chin. "How old were you when you kissed him?"

"Gosh. I must have been six, I guess. My mother had just gone, and I was feeling particularly lonely. Why?"

"Well, that explains it, of course. You weren't old enough. A princess has to be seeking true love when she kisses an enchanted frog prince. You could try again, perhaps?"

Rashpewkin hopped up on a third chair that appeared next to the table and, leaning towards Priscilla, puckered up.

She backed away. "Yuck. I don't want to kiss YOU. I mean, sorry, Rashpewkin. No offense, but we're friends now. It'd be like kissing my brother, if I had one. Besides, I'm a married woman."

Freda flicked her hand and a string of shooting stars shot across the air above them. "If you're married, it wouldn't work. Same problem. Not true love."

Rashpewkin hopped from the chair and off into the darkness. In a moment Priscilla heard his tongue snap out, followed by his grunting appreciation of the taste of some insect he'd swallowed. The sound of his hopping resumed, fading as he went deeper into the darkness.

"Don't get lost," she called out to him.

"Oh don't worry," the sorceress said. "He's bound to you by your kiss. He can wander off a bit, but he'll always find his way back."

"He's certainly handy to have around. Speaking of curses, do you know what's going on with the weather? Someone told me this drought is the result of some sorcerer's sadistic spell."

Freda fluttered her fingers and her magic globe again did its show, this time settling onto a landscape – a dark swampy area where strange figures danced around a wooden stick. Priscilla watched in fascination as the creatures spun and tumbled, sometimes losing an arm or a foot, the liberated piece dancing on its own a few beats before hopping back on.

"What kind of creatures are those?" the princess asked.

"That, my dear, is the Zone of the Zany Zombies. They've captured Edgar the Evil's wonderful wooden weather wand, and that's why your kingdom is suffering from this terrible drought. If you want the rain back in the Kingdom of the Mystic Forest, you're going to have to get the wand back."

Priscilla stared into the globe, watching the weird creatures wiggle and wobble. "Are they dangerous?"

"Well, that depends," the fairy replied. "Are you warm blooded?"

"Yes, of course."

"Then, yes, they're quite dangerous. You'll need magic to defeat the zombies. Here." She snapped her fingers and a milky glass ball appeared in her hand. "Take this with you."

Priscilla picked up the glass ball, its icy surface stinging her palm. "What is it?" When she didn't receive an answer she looked up and saw that Freda had fallen back to sleep. This time when Priscilla kicked at her, the fairy simply faded away.

"Well, I guess we'll find out," Priscilla said to Rashpewkin, and dropped the ball into her purse. "Let's head out."

They'd just reached the tent flap when they heard Freda's voice. "Look just outside my tent for a parting gift."

Chapter Four:
The Story of the Zany Zombies

A tall strand of clover lay outside the tent. When Priscilla scanned it, her attention was drawn to one of the clovers with a slightly different color. Reaching down she plucked it and saw that it had four leaves instead of the usual three. She touched it to her cheek and felt it pulsing with magic.

Turning back around, she stuck her head inside the tent, intending to thank Freda. Instead of the large room she'd just left, she discovered just an ordinary tent, empty, and only about six-feet across. "Very strange," she muttered, backing out again.

Priscilla and Rashpewkin found Boy Blue leaning on a nearby tree, polishing his instrument with his bandana. He pulled the bugle to his lips and blew a short riff that drew the princess and troll to him like fleas to a warthog.

Lowering the bugle, Blue asked, "Learn anything from the fairy?" He resumed with the bugle, burnishing its bright brass brilliant.

"Yes, indeed. We're on our way back to the castle to plan a trip. Well, after we do some shopping. I wouldn't want to come all the way to town and return empty handed. Come along, Blue. Besides Goldilocks's magic pot, you can carry my other packages, too."

She shopped among the tables on the square and in the stores of the village. By the time she was ready to head back to the castle, Boy Blue nearly staggered with the load. She'd bought packages of clothes and sweets for the Rhyme kids, a basket of her father's and husband's favorite foods for Coretta to prepare, and, oh, the LOVELIEST blue sapphire brooch.

The threesome started back along the path towards the castle, Rashpewkin bounding in front of the other two for a bit before finding something interesting on the side of the road. He'd hang about there, or just off the path into the fields or woods, until Priscilla and Blue meandered past. After they'd gotten a score of paces ahead, he'd bounce back up in front of them. At one point Priscilla saw him pick up a turtle that had the number "2" painted on its back. The creature pulled in its head and limbs until Rashpewkin set it back on the ground. The reptile stretched out its limbs and headed again on its journey down the road towards the village.

As they walked, Priscilla asked Blue about his past.

"Sad story, I'm afraid. Once I was happily married to a beautiful woman with raven hair and the face of an angel. One day I came back home to find a note on the mantle. She had heard her grandmother was ill and decided to take a picnic basket to her somewhere in the Mystic Forest. After waiting a week, I searched for her, but not a trace could be found. I was so heartbroken, I joined the army."

"Wow, that IS a sad story. And you've never heard a word?"

"There have been all types of rumors. Some say she was eaten by a wolf. One fellow swore he spotted her wandering deep in the Mystic Forest, basket still in hand. I keep looking, but no luck so far."

They walked a bit in silence until they reached a stream where they stopped for a drink. As they rested a mother duck swam by, leading her brood of six pretty yellow ducklings and one that didn't look at all like the rest of the family. It was quite ugly in fact.

When they got up to continue their walk, Blue asked again about the interview with Freda.

Priscilla replied with her own question. "What do you know of the Zone of the Zany Zombies?"

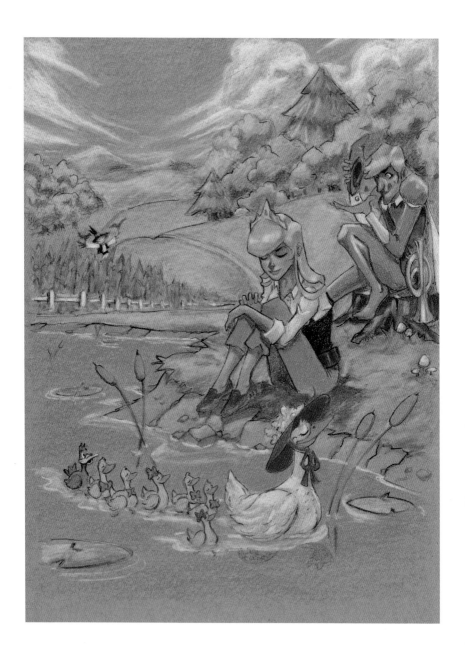

"The Zany Zombies?" Boy Blue rubbed his chin. "What business would a nice girl like you have with the Zany Zombies?"

"Well, Freda said to end the drought I've got to go to the Zone of the Zany Zombies to retrieve Edgar the Evil's wonderful wooden weather wand."

"Oh? Is THAT all?" Blue sat down on a tree stump, dropping the princess's belongings in a pile beside him. "Just waltz right in, grab the wand, and, waving sweetly at the zombies, stroll right out. Is that your plan?"

"That's the general idea, yeah. Why not?"

Blue reached down and took off one of his boots, turning it upside down and shaking out a small pea. He picked it up and examined it. "Hmm, I think this would go well under a princess's mattress some day." He dropped it into his bag.

"Tell me about the zombies, please."

He put his boot back on and stretched. Picking a dried fruit from his shoulder bag, he took a bite before offering it to Priscilla. She shook her head, and he finished it off before answering.

"The Zany Zombies were accidentally created by Edgar the Evil a few months ago. He needed some toadstools found exclusively in a monkey graveyard for one of his spells. When he got to the spot, the fungi weren't big enough. He cast a spell to encourage their growth, but messed it up. Instead of the mushrooms growing, a dozen monkey zombies sprang up from the graves. Edgar ran away so fast he dropped his wonderful wooden weather wand. Now the Zany Zombies have made it into a totem pole. By licking the pole each day, they stay undead."

"So how is that causing the drought?" Priscilla asked.

"The zombies are licking all the moisture out of the wand, and that's drying up the skies."

Priscilla scanned the fields on either side of the road. Her once verdant kingdom was turning into a land of famine. In the middle of one shriveled corn patch stood a scarecrow on a pole. A teenage girl in a gingham dress helped him down to the yellow brick road there, and he broke into a dance as the girl's black terrier barked.

Turning back to Blue, the princess stamped her foot. "We have to get it back. Let's try the simple approach. We just go in and grab the wand. What could be so hard about that?"

"What could be so hard about that?" Boy Blue scoffed. "Zombies feed on warm-blooded creatures, and you, my pretty princess, are about as warm-blooded as I've ever seen. There's no way you're going to get within a stone's throw of those creatures and survive."

Priscilla and Blue turned to the sound of a rabbit rushing

pell-mell towards them, zigging and zagging with each hop. He came to a stop at their feet, panting and peddling one leg.

"Good morning, Your Highness," the rabbit said, twitching his ears in greeting.

She curtsied in return. "A talking rabbit? Are you enchanted?"

"Maybe a little. Peter Cottontail's the name." He squeaked in dismay at the sight of Rashpewkin bouncing towards him.

"Rabbit!" Rashpewkin shouted.

"Leave it," the princess ordered, shaking her finger at him. He backed off, but kept his eyes on the creature.

The rabbit turned back to the princess. "Say, have you seen a turtle going this way?" he asked. "We're supposed to be racing, you see. I was way ahead so I thought I could take it easy. On the route I bumped into this cute little bunny I know. Guess I got a little distracted. I've always said, 'There's nothing like a little cottontail to make a guy happy.' Now I'm wondering where that darn turtle has gotten to."

Rashpewkin pointed down the road. "Went that-away."

"Thanks," the hare said, and, making a wide circle around the troll, hopped on down the road.

Priscilla indicated for Blue to pick up her packages and continue their trip. As they walked, she asked, "You have a magical bugle. Why not toot those zombies away?"

Boy Blue shook his head. "My bugle powers only work on living creatures, not on the undead."

"Well, we're going to have to get that wand. And you're going to help."

"What?" Blue stopped, lowering the bags to the ground again. Raising his palms to his forehead he murmured, "Chasing zombies was not what I had in mind as a cushy job at the castle."

Priscilla pointed at the countryside. "See those withered stalks and bone-skinny cows? Without the wonderful wooden weather wand, we'll all starve."

Blue pulled out his polka-dot bandana and wiped the dust off his bugle. He took a deep breath and brought the instrument to his lips. A deep-toned dirge poured out, sailing across the fields like an osprey over the sea. When the sounds hit the forest at the farm's edge, a couple of deer stepped out, drawn by the tune. He melded his melody towards a happy refrain, and continued on to an inspiring march. The last few bars reverted back into the lament, the final sound creating an ache in Priscilla's heart.

He slung his bugle back over his shoulder and gave the princess a wink. "I guess a man has to do what's right … at least every now and then. Very well, Highness, you can count me in. Who else will be going on this expedition?"

"My husband and my father, of course. They are Knights of the Mystic Forest, and Knights of the Mystic Forest never fail on their quests. It's in the bylaws or something. When we get back to the castle, I'll call a meeting of the Knights of the Mystic Forest and get Dad and Hector geared up for the fight."

"A site of mighty fighting knights, huh? Will they be eager to help?"

The princess called out to Rashpewkin, who had wandered off the road in chase of a butterfly. "Hey Pewker, you think the king and prince will be eager to march off on a quest?"

Rashpewkin hopped back, plucking butterfly wings out from his teeth. "King want go on quest? Do dragons blow fire?"

Priscilla patted him on the head. "Ha ha. Yes, of course they'll want to go. But … just in case, we better soften them up."

The troll looked up at her hopefully. "Mead? Lots of mead? Rashpewkin like mead."

"Yes, plenty of mead and perhaps an enticing tune by our new friend."

Chapter Five: The Knights of the Mystic Forest

Priscilla looked over at her husband, Prince Hector, sitting next to her, holding a mug of mead in each hand. His purple hair ran in a line from his scalp all the way down his back, a whole-body Mohawk left over from his days as a dragon. He stood, towering nearly seven-feet tall, and raised his two mugs. "To the king!" he shouted.

Blue had settled into a chair across the table from Priscilla. At the toast he stood and raised his mug. "To King Goethe, the wise ruler of our fair land."

The king, at the head of the table, wore his jewel-encrusted golden crown on top of his silver hair, his face boasting a full white beard. A happy smile stretched out his rosy cheeks. He stood and raised his mug, too. "Thank you, my loyal royal toiling knights. A toast to me and the kingdom."

The three clanked their mugs together, drank their mead, and sat back down. Rashpewkin hurried over and refilled the four mugs from a small barrel he dragged to the table.

Priscilla glanced over at the big grandfather clock, watching a mouse run up its side. The clock struck once, and down it ran again. Rashpewkin jumped over and made a grab for it, though he missed, and it scampered into a crack in the floorboard. "Rats," he said.

Blue said, "No, mice." He pointed to a corner where three of the rodents seemed to be wandering around at random. "Try getting those," he suggested. "Those three are blind."

Rashpewkin rushed over, swinging a carving knife. He managed to cut off one of their tails, but otherwise the three rodents escaped inside the grandfather clock. He gobbled down the tail.

"Okay, Dad," the princess said. "If you've loosened your tongue enough, perhaps we can talk about the zombies, huh?"

"All in good time, my princess. As King of the Realm of the Mystic Forest, I hereby declare this meeting of the Knights of the Table of the Mystic Kingdom called to order. Knights, sound off!"

The prince stood again, banging his head on the rafter, showering dirt into the room. He laughed loudly, pushing the cracked and sagging rafter back into place. Raising a thumb in an "up" sign, Hector announced, "Prince Hector, sworn to your service, my liege."

King Goethe looked over at Blue and indicated for him to rise.

"Uh. I'm Boy Blue," he said. "I'm, well, gosh. Does this mean I'm a knight now?"

"Yes, yes, of course," the king replied. "With all the duties of such an honorific title. You must be honorable, so each evening we can say to you 'Good Knight.'"

"Great," Priscilla said. "So, now that we've had roll call, about those zombies …"

"First we must sing our anthem," King Goethe interrupted. He and Hector boomed out the words as Blue mumbled along.

We are the Knights of the Mystic Forest Kingdom.

Adventurers all are we.

We'll seek the fight and win the goods

For honor, joy, and pageantry."

Hector and Goethe hooked elbows and did a swing around each other. Falling into their chairs, they downed their mugs and held them up for Rashpewkin to refill. The king stroked his white beard, twirling some of the hairs into knots. Pointing up at the banners on the wall, he named off the quests each one commemorated: *the Quest of the Oblivious Ogres, the Quest of the Wicked Weasels, the Quest of the Wacky Wombats,* and so forth. After the naming of each one, Hector and Blue yelled, "Hip Hip Hooray!" and all three took a slug of their mead.

"I'm going to like this Knight business," Blue said, wiping off some lingering mead from his lips with his sleeve. He held out his mug for Rashpewkin to refill.

"So, it seems my brave knights are ready for another quest, huh Dad?"

Goethe turned to his daughter, worry lines creasing his forehead. "These quests aren't to be taken lightly, my dear. You'll have to stay here and keep the kingdom under control, of course."

She stood and stomped her foot. "No Siree Bob! This is MY quest idea, and you're not going to leave me behind."

"But quests can be dangerous," the king insisted.

Hector reached across the table and took Priscilla's hand. "My amazing wife! If she wants to come, I say she should come."

The king looked at Blue, who just shrugged.

"Well…." The king plucked a June bug out of his beard and watched it fly out the window. "I suppose we should take her. And lots of magic, too. How are we set up for magic?" This he directed towards Priscilla.

"I picked up a few magical items from town." She pulled the glass ball given to her by Freda the Fair Fairy and tossed it to her father. He caught it, taking a quick look before handing it over to Hector, who tossed it to Blue. He placed it on the table, and all three men blew on their palms.

"Yow! That's cold," one said.

"So what does it do?" another asked.

Priscilla picked it up. A slight bluish color twirled through the whiteness, and, though it was cold in her hand, it clearly wasn't as chilly in her hands as in the men's. "Don't know. It's magical, for sure."

Blue cleared his throat. "Ahem. How do you propose we approach the Zone of the Zany Zombies? You know, those crazy dead monkeys eat out the brains of anyone who goes near them." He put his bugle to his lips and sounded out the first few bars of "Taps."

Hector stood up, knocking the rafter again. He pounded his chest with his fist. "Hector not afraid."

Priscilla stood and leaned into his chest. "Oh, my brave, strong husband!" She squeezed his bulging arm muscle, sighing with delight.

King Goethe nodded. "Be purposefully pertinacious, buoyant boy." Turning to Blue, he said, "You boast of boogie-woogie bounty, so, brightly boisterous Blue, don't be baleful or bitter. Rather be benevolent and beneficial. Joyfully join our Quest for the Zany Zombies."

The bugler shrugged. "I guess I'll come along and see how you manage to mangle and manhandle the miscreants."

"Ha! That's the spirit. Together we'll smite those slithering slathering scrappy simians," the king proclaimed.

"We'll pulverize those pitiful prattling primates," Hector added.

"We'll … um …" Blue took another mead sip. "We'll apprehend the abominable acrobatic apes.

"Hurrah!" Priscilla called. "We'll squash those supernatural soulless specters!"

The king turned to Rashpewkin. "You, Troll. Go tell Coretta to prepare three days of rations for the five of us. Have Blackburn prepare four steeds, and I suppose you'll be wanting a jack-ass. We'll leave in an hour."

"What?" Priscilla shouted. "Tonight? Why can't we wait for the morning sun?"

"The Zone of the Zany Zombies is just over a day's ride. If we get a start now, and an early start tomorrow, we can be in-the-zone before nightfall tomorrow."

The three men stood, clanked their cups together and paused, all looking at Priscilla. Giving a happy smile, she held her mug out to Rashpewkin. After he filled it, she clanked the others hard enough to splash juice onto her husband's face. He licked it off with his long forked tongue, another dragon leftover.

"To the Quest of the Zany Zombies!" they shouted.

Leaving the others to have "one last round," Priscilla went up to her bedroom to prepare. Though she'd once been into the Mystic Forest seeking a wizard, she'd never been on a quest before. She chose two dresses, some pants and tops, and a handful of underthings, enough to go four days she figured. In a separate bag she packed some of her jewelry, the four-leaf clover, and Freda's glass ball. Stuffing in a third bag containing her toiletries, she made her way downstairs to join the others.

She found Rashpewkin relaxing on the drawbridge, his feet hanging over the moat and a big smile across his face.

"What's got you so happy?" she asked him.

"Found grasshopper and ant arguing," he said. "Ant say work good. Grasshopper say play better."

"Oh? Did you settle the argument?"

"Yep. Eat 'em both."

Priscilla looked up at the sound of horses to find that

Blackburn, the castle blacksmith, had brought four horses and a donkey up from the stables. He proceeded to secure everyone's luggage onto the beasts. Prince Hector came over and lifted Priscilla onto her steed, a good-size red creature with a blue ribbon tied in a bow around his neck. The horse tossed his head, calming when Priscilla leaned forward and stroked him. "Seems like a gentle horse. What's his name?"

"Fireball," King Goethe answered, coming up and patting the horse, too. "Don't worry, my dear. Fireball is very mild as long as you stroke him. Otherwise he gets frightened. He's very fearful of small rodents."

"And big cats," Hector added.

"And birds," Blackburn said.

"And lightning," Coretta added, coming up with the food.

Everyone in turn began adding …

"Moon shadows."

"His own shadow."

"The sound of water."

"The sound of wind."

"The sound of people's voices."

"The sound of song."

"And of laughter."

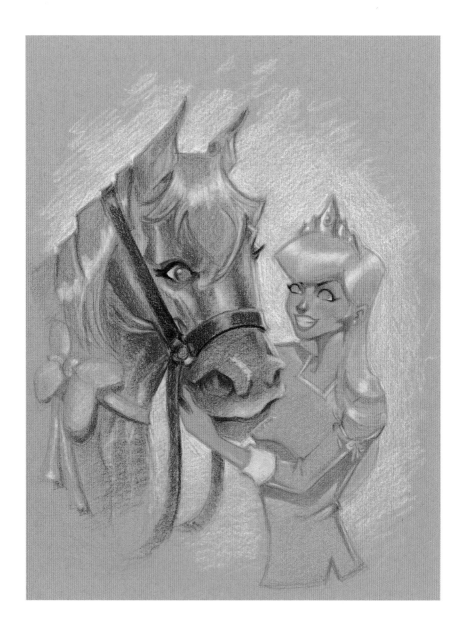

"Flower aromas."

"And clover's color."

"And so," the king finished, "you should have nothing to worry about." He climbed onto his own steed, a large white horse with a patch over one eye. The horse turned and took a nip at Fireball's haunch, causing the red horse to tremble and shy away.

Hector and Blue mounted their horses, too, while Rashpewkin sprang lightly onto the back of his donkey. With a few final instructions to the castle staff, King Goethe raised his sword high in the air.

"Knights of the Mystic Forest, we are off on a Quest. We go for greater glory and gracious goodness. Ready all?"

They all shouted, "READY!"

With a blast from Blue's bugle, they sallied forth down the path into the Mystic Forest.

Chapter Six:
Traveling through the
Mystic Forest

Dipping under the verdant canopy of the Mystic Forest trees brought them into another world. Birds serenaded them from nests high above. Mammals with long prehensile tails hung from branches just beyond the travelers' reach. Colorful hand-sized fragrant flowers decorated vines hanging in lazy loops from every tree.

Priscilla, with Rashpewkin riding by her side, followed Prince Hector and King Goethe in the lead, with Blue taking the rear guard. She kept a careful watch on the woods, spying the flurry of little creatures with their wide eyes watching from every side. A butterfly family hovered near her ears for a few minutes before wavering away into the shadows. Priscilla stroked her horse periodically, which kept

Fireball calm, without any problems from the strange sights, sounds, and smells around them.

Priscilla noticed the shadows deepening as the sun neared its bedtime. Although she felt safe enough with all the men around, still this WAS the Mystic Forest, and who knew what kind of strange animals would show up? She was just about to call out to ask her father when they would stop, when the path opened up onto a small clearing. From the trees along the edges, flowers hung like wallpaper. A stream gurgled out of some rocks on one edge and a lovely apple tree in the middle offered plump red fruit.

Hector pulled off the camping gear and went hunting while Blue set up the tents and supplies. The king took care of the horses, sending Rashpewkin off to gather wood for the fire pit. After going through the rations and making dinner preparations, Priscilla decided to pick some of the apples to add to their meal.

She plucked the first one and was about to put it into her bag when she heard a hiss. Turning sharply, she jumped back at the sight of a thick orange and black striped serpent.

"Isss it the Prin-cessss?"

She took another step back. "Oh! Well, yes, that's me. Who are you?"

"Sssome sssay I'm ssserpent. Sssome sssay I'm ssssome thing

elsssse. Isss that your sssscrumptiousss apple?"

Priscilla glanced in the direction of his vision, the apple in her hand. "Well … I mean, it's a wild tree, right? Perfectly good apples?" She tried to look at the snake when she talked, but each time she caught sight of his eyes she began feeling hypnotized, so she stared at the apple instead.

"Yesss. Itsss sssafe. Perfectly sssafe."

She started to take a bite and stopped. "What do you mean, safe? What would it do to me?"

"Ssso sssupicccciousss sssisster?" The snake wound himself back up on his branch, flexing his muscles hard enough for her to hear the branch crack. He flung himself to a limb closer to her, grabbing it with his tail, and flopping down within a foot of her face. "Yesss. Isss do sssomething. Isss make you wissse. Isss wanting wisssdom isss you?"

She brought up the apple, again stopping just before it reached her mouth. "That's all there is to it? I'd be smarter? What could be wrong with that?"

"Yesss. Princesss be sssmarter. Ssshe isss biting?"

Priscilla looked into the snake's face, his big green eyes pulsating into her brain. "Consssume," he hissed.

She lifted the apple to her mouth, just lowering her teeth to

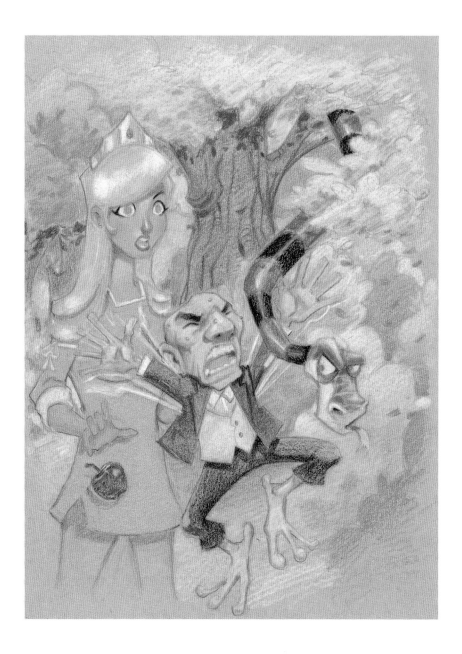

its skin when Rashpewkin leaped up and knocked it away.

"Bad! Bad Serpent! Go away! Shoo! Shoo!" He jumped up and down, waving his arms wildly. He scooped up a rock with his foot and threw it at the snake. The snake slithered away hissing.

Priscilla shook herself out of the trance. "What was that all about?"

Rashpewkin held up the apple. Pointing to two small holes, he said, "Snake poison apple. See fang marks?"

He was about to throw it away when Priscilla took it from his hands and dropped it into her purse. "This just might come in handy." She reached up and picked four more apples, studying them each carefully for marks. Finding none, she brought them, in a separate bag, back to the camp.

There she helped Rashpewkin prepare some small mammals Hector had caught, and soon the stew pot sat over the welcoming fire, boiling their dinner.

"There's nothing like an evening around a campfire," Boy Blue mused, as the five of them relaxed beside the fire pit. "Who knows a story?"

Prince Hector spoke up. "I'll tell you the tale of how I became a dragon. I grew up in the land of a thousand lakes, making my living as a lumberjack. I swung a huge ax and loaded the felled trees on my blue ox to pull to market. Well, one day a dragon came to our land. His fire breath burned the woods we needed to live on, and he talked non-stop – jabbered so much we called him Jabberwocky. Someone had to do something, so my grandfather sent me off to kill the dragon. He let me use his favorite blade, the magical Vorpal sword."

Hector stood and demonstrated, pulling out his sword and taking swings at some hanging vines, sending their leaves showering down upon them.

"I found the dragon hiding in his crystal cave, sitting on his hoard of treasure, looking quite smaug, er, smug. My blade went snicker-snack, and, though I did succeed in killing the beast, in the process he bit me, turning me into a dragon, too – a bit embarrassing for the love interest."

He settled back down on his bedroll, and Priscilla cuddled up next to him, stroking his chest. "So tell me, Dear. What made you think you could come to me and find a wife?"

"I had heard from several of the knights who came to try to slay me that you were looking for a strong brave husband." He leaned over and kissed her on the forehead. "They said you were a pip, and, by Merlin's beard, you're a positively poppingly picturesque pip, beautiful, smart, brave … someday we're going to raise a parcel of little knights and knightesses. Pointing up to the tree boughs he said, "Look up there. It's a baby cradle. Maybe it's a portent of some kind."

Priscilla looked at the treetops and spotted the cradle. A strong wind picked up, and the cradle rocked and rocked, and, with a crack, its branch broke, bringing the cradle, baby and all, plummeting to the earth. She screamed.

Blue, who had been leaning against the tree trunk, stepped forward and caught the cradle. He set it on the ground and pulled back the cover. A strange green creature stared up at him. It hopped out of the cradle and shuffled its big frog-like feet in the dirt, looking around at the group. Standing about two-feet tall, the creature had big floppy ears on either side of a bulging-eyed warty face. She wore a cute pink bonnet and a pink skirt with large white polka dots.

Hector took up his sword and brought its tip a smidgen away from the thing's nose. "Who be ye, oh fearsome creature," he shouted. "Friend or foe?"

"Ribbet?"

"Ah, playing dumb, are ye?" Hector raised his sword above the creature's head. "We can slice and dice you in mere moments. I imagine you'll make a delicious soup."

"Ribbet?"

Priscilla watched the creature's eyes grow ever wider, blowing up to balloon size. The princess reached up and placed her hand on her husband's arm. "Stop now, Love. She's clearly just a harmless frog."

Rashpewkin, who had been off on a short reconnaissance, hopped out of the woods and bounced over to the green thing. "Hurrah! Hurrah! Look who it be! Looky, looky!" He hopped in a circle around the big bullfrog who looked at Rashpewkin with bewilderment.

"You know this amphibian, do you?" Priscilla asked.

"Righty, righty! This be my cousin, Jeri-Myah! Remember? Fairy Freda enchant both."

Blue scratched his chin. "I seem to remember stories about Jeri-Myah the Bullfrog. Does she drink a mighty fine wine?"

"Ribbet?" The frog looked from one to the other.

"What's wrong with her?" Priscilla asked. "At least you could talk to me when I first found you."

"Magic wears out," the troll explained. "Got Magic?" he asked, licking the white foam off his lips.

King Goethe shrugged. "Not me. I have a few leprechaun duggets and my beard brush." Blue and Hector both shook their heads.

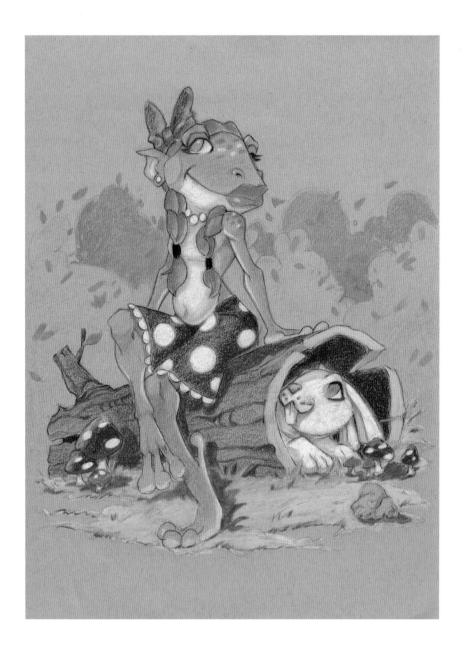

Priscilla dug through her purse and brought out the four-leaf clover. "How about this?"

Jeri-Myah shot out her long tongue and snagged the clover from the princess's hand, pulling it in and making a big display of swallowing it, her throat puffing up to her jaw line and all the way down to her stomach as the wad worked its way down. A greenish glow emanated from her belly, working its way down to her webbed feet and up to her forehead. She gave a big burp.

"Ah, that be better!" she exclaimed. "Thanky." She stretched and twisted a bit, raising one foot and staring at her toes as they wiggled. She reached out and grabbed Rashpewkin in both arms, bringing him in for a hug. "Hi-dee-doo, cousin. Where you be go?"

Rashpewkin swept his arm to indicate his companions. "These be Mystic Forest Knights. We be off on great quest! You come too?"

"You off to see Wizard?"

"No, Zany Zombies."

Jeri-Myah nodded. "Okee-dokey. Them zombies monkey 'round."

Rubbing their big-smiled cheeks up against each other, Jeri-Myah and Rashpewkin hugged one more time. Holding each other's hands, they hopped off to a nearby pond.

Late into the moonlit night, as Priscilla snuggled against her husband, she heard them croaking to each other. She thought, *no doubt catching up on lost time. What a lucky find. Gee, everything is going so well on this quest. Now, if we can only figure out how to get past those zombies to get the wonderful wooden weather wand all will be swell.*

Chapter Seven: The Hut of Candy

Priscilla awoke to the sounds of Rashpewkin's and Jeri-Myah's chatter. Around her the forest birds produced a symphony. The morning flowers sprayed a perfume cloud. She reached over, placing her hand on Hector's empty sleeping bag. It still held a hint of his body heat.

She sat up, brushing the hair out of her face. A dozen yards away, Rashpewkin and Jeri-Myah huddled at the campfire, the two of them taking turns with their long tongues snagging insects drawn to the flames.

"Hey, Pewker," she called out.

Rashpewkin gave her a long-armed wave. "Goodee morning, Princess P."

She waved back and, surveying the empty bags, asked, "What happened to the boys?"

"They go hunting. Tell Rashpewkin they be back pronto."

Priscilla carried her towel and a change of clothes upstream a bit. Just as she felt she had gone far enough, she came upon a pussycat pushing a pea-green boat into the stream. Sitting in the bow was a large owl that said, "Whooo are youuu?"

"I'm Princess Priscilla, of course." Holding her hand to her mouth, she tried to suppress her laugh. "Please excuse me, but, goblin globules, what a strange sight the two of you make!"

The cat gave her a cold cat's eye and said, "Purr-mit me. We Purr-fur to be alone." She gave the boat a push into the water, made a leap to land right inside, and quickly the current took them away. Just before they dropped out of sight, the princess saw the owl pull out a guitar and begin to sing.

She washed out the clothes she'd worn the day before. As they dried, she washed herself thoroughly, giving special attention to her hair, which seemed to have adopted a family of gnats.

Returning to camp, she found the two green creatures standing around the fire, each taking a turn to stare into the kettle suspended above it.

"What's for breakfast? I don't smell anything cooking." She

peered into the pot, seeing water bubbling slowly. "No breakfast?"

Rashpewkin looked up with knitted brow. "Prince promise bring back food. No return yet."

She gazed up towards the sun, now a good bit above the tree line. Figuring she'd been up for over an hour, she wondered why the men hadn't returned. An elk stepped into the clearing and gave her a snort. Seeing she wasn't going to put up a fight, it took a long drink from the stream before disappearing back into the woods.

"I knew we should have packed more food. Last night the boys ate up almost everything Coretta sent us off with." Picking an apple off the tree she munched on it as she peered into the woods. "I wonder what's taking them so long. You think they got into trouble?"

Rashpewkin hopped up next to her and placed his hand at his brow mimicking her. He, too, stared into the woods. "Rashpewkin think Mystic Woods have big magic. Royal Knights find big trouble."

Priscilla remembered some of the stories she'd heard about the Mystic Forest, the weird creatures and magical beings. "Well," she said to Rashpewkin, "we better go find them."

Instructing Jeri-Myah to stay at the camp, Priscilla followed her pet troll as he tracked the men on the route they took into the forest. He had little trouble following the broken branches and footprints in the mud, and, within a quarter hour, they reached the edge of a clearing.

"There!"

The men's footsteps led to the front door of a little cottage made all of candy. Its gingerbread walls sported bright colored gumdrops, the roof dripped with thick white frosting, and the garden's fence consisted of giant-size candy corns. On top, a chimney of peanut brittle emitted a thin wisp of smoke.

"House look friendly," Rashpewkin said. "Nourishing, too!" He hopped into the clearing and up to the candy cane fence, where he began nibbling on one edge. "Good!"

"I don't know about this." The princess came beside him, but didn't take a bite. "Looks suspicious to me."

Rashpewkin shrugged and continued eating. In a minute or two he stopped and stood staring.

"Rashpewkin?" Priscilla reached over and shook his shoulder. "Hey, are you okay?"

She turned to the sound of the door opening. On the porch stood a lovely, thin, tall woman with flowing black hair and skin color to match.

"Ah, visitors," she said, her voice musical and mystifying. "Do come in." She beckoned with a wave of her hand.

Rashpewkin took one step towards her, and Priscilla held

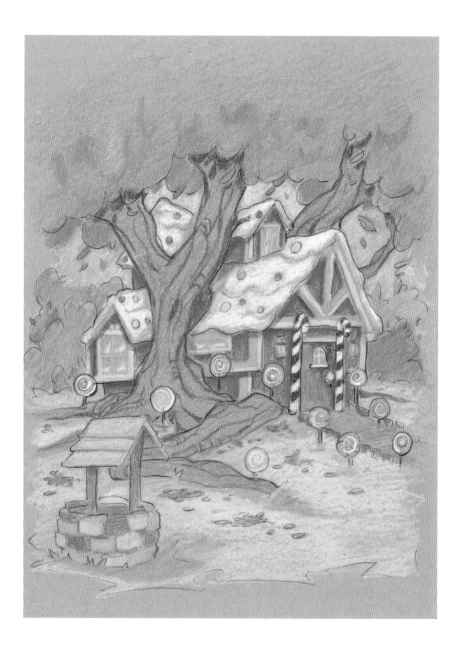

him back by his shoulder.

"Who are you?" she asked.

The tall woman gave a wicked smile. "Oh, just a poor peasant woman, living a lonely life in a small humble cottage. I'm so delighted to have visitors. Please, have a bite of my home. As your little troll has found, it's all quite delicious."

Priscilla turned Rashpewkin to look into his face. His eyes held an empty stare, as if he were sleepwalking. She shook him without effect.

Turning back to the witch, for that, she decided, was what the woman must be, Priscilla shook her head. "No thank you. I'm not hungry at the moment. By the way, allow me to introduce myself. I'm Princess Priscilla."

The witch gave a wry smile. "Ah, yes. Even in this far corner of the Mystic Forest I've heard of you and ..." She looked over at Rashpewkin. "Your troll." Holding her head erect, she announced, "My name is Samantha Stevens. You may call me Sam."

"Well, Sam. I'm looking for my family. My father, husband, and a friend seem to have gotten lost. Have you seen them?"

"Hmm. Three men, you say?" The witch rubbed her chin. "No, not sure I've seen them."

"That's strange. Their footsteps lead right up to your cottage."

The tall woman beckoned with her hand again. "You're welcome to come in and look around. Perhaps you'll be hungry when you get inside. Bring your troll too."

Priscilla let loose of Rashpewkin's shoulder, and the troll hopped past the witch and into the cottage. The princess followed him, stopping just outside the door. She squinted into the dark room, lit only by some red coals glowing in the fireplace. Before Priscilla's vision could adjust, Sam shoved her inside, jumped in after her, and slammed and locked the door.

Priscilla spotted King Goethe, Prince Hector, Boy Blue, and Rashpewkin standing in one corner, staring with blank looks. With a glance she saw the rest of the little home consisted of a dining table set for one, a bed in one corner, and a small kitchen with sink, cutting board, and a rack holding a half dozen large gleaming knifes.

"There they are," the princess said, pointing to her family and friend. "I thought you said you hadn't seen them."

Sam shrugged. "Oh, THOSE men. Well, they don't talk much, you see. And, anyway, I'm planning on having them for dinner. You will join me, of course?"

"You're planning on killing the men and eating them?" Priscilla raced back to the door and tried to jiggle the lock loose, but it wouldn't budge. She looked around and saw that, except for the chimney, the room had no other openings.

"Well, I'd prefer some fruit and vegetables," Sam said with a sigh. "But, as you can see, my garden only grows candy, so I have to live on what I can catch. You sure you won't join me? I'm thinking of starting with an arm from the big guy. It's clearly quite meaty."

Priscilla reached into her bag and brought out the serpent's apple. "You say you'd prefer some fruit? How about this delicious apple?"

The sorceress stared at it, her eyes wide. "Oh! That looks wonderful! Please, oh yes, I'd like that apple. What do you want for it?"

"We'll talk about that in a moment. Enjoy." Priscilla handed her the fruit.

Sam took a big bite. At first nothing seemed to happen, and she chewed thoughtfully. Once she swallowed, though, the witch's eyes began glowing. She moaned and spun around. The front door flew open and the fireplace roared with a bright flame.

"What have you done, you nasty little girl?" the witch demanded. "You've poisoned me!"

"Nonsense. It's just an apple of wisdom."

Sam moaned again. "Oh, the apple has taught me the difference between good and evil, and now I realize how bad I've been." She waved her hand in the direction of the men, and they all came alert. Hector rushed over to the wall, and, taking down a knife, raised it to strike down the witch.

Priscilla grabbed his arm and stopped him. "Don't. She's okay now."

Sam walked outside and they all followed, taking deep breaths of the fresh air – a relief from the smoky stale air in the cottage. Priscilla came up to Sam and placed a hand on her shoulder. She saw that Sam was crying.

Through her tears, the witch said, "I've been so bad, so very, very bad."

"It's okay; you didn't know any better," Priscilla held out her arms, and the witch came into them for a hug. The princess patted her gently on the back.

"What can I ever do to redeem myself?" Sam asked.

"Well, we're on a quest to get Edgar's wonderful wooden weather wand back from the Zany Zombies. Do you think you could help?"

The sorceress's brow furrowed. "Hmm. I don't know anything about them. But I know who would. Along your route there's a stone obelisk that knows everything. It always deals squarely with those who ask it one question."

Priscilla thanked her. Signaling to Rashpewkin, who'd gathered up a handful of candy to take with him, the five of them headed back to the campsite to continue their journey.

Chapter Eight: The Stone Obelisk

Narrow pine trees made up this part of the forest, their tall canopy and bare lower branches creating an open, easily traveled landscape. A temperate breeze drifted in the air, keeping them cool. Once a bear rumbled across the path ahead of them, and a bit later they passed a family of wide-eyed deer watching them go by.

Riding in the lead, King Goethe kept them headed in the proper direction. Priscilla was surprised at how well he knew the Mystic Forest. She wondered how many times he'd been through it in his many years as king. Dozens?

He held up his hand, bringing the group to a stop next to a woman in a red hooded jacket leaning against a tree. In her hand she held a large curved-tail basket covered by an embroidered cloth.

She curtsied. "Good morning, Your Highness. It's good to see you again. What brings you to this far corner of the Mystic Forest this morning?"

He climbed off his horse and shook her hand. "Miss Hood, it's good to see you again, too." He swept his hand behind him to indicate his group. "We're off on a Quest. There's my daughter, Princess Priscilla, followed by her husband, Prince Hector. Behind the donkey with the two creatures, rides my Royal Bugler, the one hiding his face."

He indicated the woman. "Quest-seekers, this is my dear subject and long time friend, Miss Red Riding Hood."

She curtsied to the group. Holding up the woven basket, she asked, "Are you hungry? I have my never-ending lunch basket. It'll be plenty to feed your group."

"Why, that's very kind of you, Red. As a matter of fact, our breakfast hunting trip was interrupted. We could stand with a bit of nourishment." King Goethe signaled for everyone to dismount, and they gathered around the young woman.

Red opened the basket and gave a roll, some cheese, and a piece of fruit to Jeri-Myah, Rashpewkin, King Goethe, and Prince Hector. When she turned to Priscilla, the princess said, "I didn't think that small basket could hold all that. Yet its just as full as when you started."

Red laughed. "Oh, there's always enough to feed everyone in the cornucopia basket." She handed Priscilla her share.

When Red turned to the last of the group, she froze. "Is it really you?" she asked.

Boy Blue gave a big smile. "Hey there, Beautiful. Long time no see."

She dropped her basket and wrapped her arms around him in a solid hug. "Why you old wolf! Where did you get off to?"

He held up his hands in a pleading motion. "Me? You were the one who disappeared. You said you went off to see your grandmother. What happened?"

"I had to nurse my grandma for several weeks while foraging for food, too. She was so poor we felt the wolf was at the door, so to speak. Anyway, when I got back you were gone. What's your story?"

Boy Blue gave her another hug before telling his story. "I had traveled to several towns looking for you. One day I was playing my bugle on a town corner. A foursome of soldiers came up each holding a mug of ale. One dropped a coin in my hat and asked me to play some military tunes. I put together a medley right there on the spot. After applauding they invited me to join them in a cup of ale. Just before we got into the tavern, they pulled me into an alley and shanghaied me. Next thing I knew, I was in the army!" He played a short burst of a military dirge before continuing his tale.

"Turned out they needed a bugle boy. Made me serve five years before I got out. I've been searching for you ever since. I checked our old hut, but you were gone and a family of three bears had moved in."

He grabbed her in a hug, and she snuggled deep into his chest.

"You two seem so happy together," Priscilla observed. "How'd you meet?"

"When Blue was younger he used to take naps under haystacks," Red said. "One day an old gnome captured me and ordered me to turn straw into gold. When I went out to the haystack to get some pieces, there Little Boy Blue was, fast asleep. When I woke him and explained my problem, he promised to help me. In no time he banished the gnome with one of his magic tunes, and I've been in love with my bugle boy ever since."

"There's nothing like true love!" Priscilla said. Hector bent down and kissed her on the forehead.

"I guess this means I won't be continuing on the Quest, your Royalties," Blue said with a bow. "I have some family time to make up."

"Quite understandable, my boy," King Goethe said. "You've done a yeoman's work, and your King thanks you. Here." He reached into his purse and brought out a handful of gold leprechaun duggets. Placing them into Boy Blue's hand, the king said, "May your lives be most wondrous fairy tales."

They all settled down to eat, and the king showed Hector how to make a sandwich from the bread and cheese. Red brought out a flask of water and poured them all full cups, and Priscilla noted the pitcher never seemed to empty either.

"What kind of quest are you off on now?" Red asked, watching them eat.

King Goethe took a large gulp from his drink before answering. "It's the Quest of the Zany Zombies, my friend. We must retrieve the wonderful wooden weather wand to save the kingdom."

"The Zany Zombies? Oh my. You mustn't go after them, your Highness. They'll eat out your brain!"

The king took another bite, swallowing before turning back to Red. "Someone told us there's a stone obelisk nearby that can tell us how to defeat the Zany Zombies. Have you heard of such a thing? Do you know where it is?"

"Indeed I do, your Highness. The stone obelisk lies just a half league due West. Be wary, for it's a treacherous beast that speaks in riddles. I bid you good fortune on your journey."

After eating, and thanking Red for the information and her generosity, they bid Boy Blue a final farewell. Remounting, the remaining five travelers rode on through the trees, soon arriving at a small clearing where stood a square obelisk. Ten-feet tall, the white-marbled, four-sided stone column seemed totally blank. They all dismounted and came up to it, Rashpewkin running his hand along the smooth marble edges and Jeri-Myah giving it a big lick.

Prince Hector put his hands on his hips and nodded approval. "This is the biggest spike I've ever seen. Bigger even than me. I wonder who built it?"

A face with black opal eyes appeared on the four sides of the obelisk. Each face spoke in unison.

> *Here in the meadow, beneath tree shadow*
> *Shrub color mages, in shiny cages*
> *Made Magic frightening, thunder and lightning,*
> *Creating me, a talking key*
> *To answer each man, if I can*
> *A single query, so be leery.*
> *Ask me once, or be a dunce*
> *The second time, I'll nary whine.*

"What does all that mean?" Prince Hector asked. However, the faces had disappeared, leaving only a smooth stone surface. He turned to the others and repeated his question.

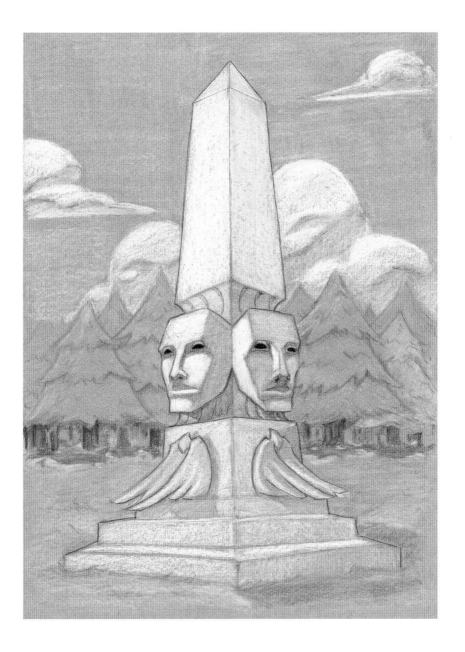

Rashpewkin hopped up. "One question. Each get one question. Me turn. Oh stone spike, listen Rashpewkin. How Rashpewkin be human again?"

The faces reappeared and chanted in unison.

> *A boy turns frog, upon a log,*
> *By enchantment strong, much prolonged*
> *'til princess's kiss, makes remiss*
> *So do not grieve, you self deceive.*
> *You've found again, your dearest friend*
> *To meet your need, to have you freed,*
> *Your search could end, if mind you bend.*
> *A kiss is best, from royal princess.*

The troll shrugged. "Rashpewkin know rules. Where Rashpewkin find another princess? One who love and kiss troll?"

The obelisk had turned back inanimate and not an answer did it give.

"Stubborn piece of stone, isn't it?" King Goethe observed.

"No wait! That wasn't my question!"

But it was too late. The faces reappeared.

> *Made to talk, we shall not balk*
> *Be it question simple, or full of dimples,*
> *Just be aware, if you dare*
> *Our answers few, always true*
> *For see our corners? Take as warners*
> *You take care, our answer's square*
> *Have some fun, but ask only one.*

Priscilla observed, "The stone talks a lot like our cook

Coretta."

Prince Hector said, "Sort of. Coretta cooks square meals and the obelisk gives square deals."

King Goethe turned to Priscilla. "Be careful, Dear. You only have one question, and we need to know how to beat the zombies."

Priscilla looked the stone tower up and down as she carefully planned her question. She took a deep breath before speaking.

"Oh great stone obelisk, he of truth telling answers, please tell us completely how we are to defeat the zombies. We must get rid of them without us getting hurt, and we must recover the wonderful wooden weather wand. What must we do, and what magic do we need?"

Once again the faces appeared, eyebrows of moss and mouth of a deep blue.

The answers you seek may make you meek.
You carry the ball and yet might fall.
For zombies eat warm-blooded meat
Yet one of you could go on through
And place the ball way up tall
For zombies to lick. Then grab the stick.
They give no peep, they fall asleep.
Rush home again, and make it rain.

Well, that seems simple enough … I think." Priscilla looked at her father and her husband. "Right?"

King Goethe scratched his chin. "Hmm, it seems to me it said one of us had to go on through and place the magic ball up high. But ... which one?"

Hector thumped his chest. "Me of course! I'm the biggest, bravest, bodacious battler that's ever been. I'll zip zap and zig zag like a super zipper and bountifully bash those Zany Zombies in their hideous heads."

Priscilla grabbed him in a hug. "Oh, you brave, brave man. But, no, it can't be you. They'll suck your brains out. I do love your body, I admit, but without your brains, how would you know to tell me how beautiful I am?"

The king said, "Of course, it has to be me. The kindly king cares considerably for favorite friendly folks." He pulled out his sword and swung it back and forth. "A swish and a swash, a jab and a jot. I'll snickersee those sickerees. With a whip and a whap, I'll swipe the wondrous wand and home we'll head."

Priscilla let loose of Hector and came over and hugged her father even tighter. "Oh no you don't, Daddy. You're the only Daddy I've ever had, and you're NOT going to sacrifice yourself to the zombies. That can't be the right answer."

Rashpewkin jumped up and down. "Rashpewkin know. Rashpewkin know."

All turned to him. "What do you know?" Priscilla asked.

"Who one."

"Who won what?"

"Who one fight zombies."

Priscilla squatted so she could be face to face. "You don't mean you? You're half frog, true, but being half human you're warm-blooded, right? You'd have to be all frog …"

As the thought occurred to her, she turned to stare at Jeri-Myah.

"Yepperee," Rashpewkin said. "She be cold-blooded. She the one."

Jeri-Myah paled. "You want me fight zombies? Me?"

The obelisk faces appeared.

> *Little one asks, and finds a task.*
> *A clearing soon, under full moon*
> *Zombies dance and zombies prance*
> *And eat the brains of their domains.*
> *But they eschew a certain crew*
> *Frogs well told, whose blood is cold.*
> *You'll make the switch, without a glitch*
> *And show the way to save the day.*

King Goethe looked up at the sun, now just above the treetops. "Yeti Yodels! We better get a move on. I had hoped to be near the Zany Zombie Zone by sunset. Now it looks like we'll be traveling into the dark. We'll get a few hours sleep and then awake before dawn for the adventure."

They mounted their steeds and continued on their quest.

Chapter Nine: The Zone of the Zany Zombies

The last glimmer of sunlight filtered through the trees when King Goethe finally called a halt. Priscilla saw he'd brought them into a small meadow edged by a stream full of fish. In the encroaching dark, the king set up the tents, Priscilla laid out the bags inside, and Hector gathered wood for the fire. Rashpewkin found some berries and mushrooms for dinner while Jeri-Myah caught five fish. Soon they settled around the campfire enjoying a delicious meal.

"The Zone of the Zany Zombies sits but another half league to our west," King Goethe said, pointing in the general direction.

Pricilla snuggled closer to her husband. "Are we safe here? They're not going to come after us, are they?"

Hector kissed her forehead. "No need to fret fair female. Brave knights through the brackish night will keep your brain nigh."

"We will arise before dawn," the king announced. "Under the full moon, Hector and I will charge into the camp with swords flashing, making fast work of those sinister zombies. You other three must stay in camp to be safe."

"Hipporree!" Rashpewkin shouted. "King and Prince be heroes!"

The two men stood and bowed, and Rashpewkin and Jeri-Myah applauded.

"Now wait a minute," Priscilla said. "I thought Jeri-Myah was the one going in."

King Goethe scoffed. "A frog? You think a frog can defeat a dozen bouncing zombies?" He unsheathed his sword and flashed it around. "Cold steel! That's all monsters can understand. Right Hector?"

The prince waved his sword, too, cutting a swank figure eight through the night air, dropping a fly buzzing to the ground. "I just took his wings off," he announced.

"You're a skilled swordsman, my darling husband. Still, didn't the obelisk say Jeri-Myah was the only one immune to the Zombies' brain thirst?"

The king scoffed. "I say again, it's cold steel that'll win the game. You'll see us return victorious, my daughter."

Settled into her sleeping bag that night, Priscilla listened to the crickets, their sounds heard between the men's snores. Her fear of what might happen in the coming battle kept her awake for hours. She had just drifted off to dreams of attacking monkeys when she felt someone shaking her shoulder.

"Wakee-wakee," Rashpewkin said. "We go hurry."

"What … what's happened?" She sat, shaking the cobwebs out of her head. A spider fell off too.

"Jeri-Myah grab ball and go bye-bye."

Priscilla changed back into her dress and pulled on her boots, hurrying to join Rashpewkin outside. He held a compass and a bag.

"This way west," he said, leading the princess into the woods.

They'd traveled only a few minutes when they heard fiendish laughter ahead. Soon they came upon Jeri-Myah crouching behind some bushes, beyond which they could make out a clearing. Rashpewkin and Priscilla joined her, and the princess took a peek through the leaves.

In a treeless area as big as two barns a dozen graves stood open, each with a stone marker. In the middle of the area a walking stick stood erect, glowing in the moon's eerie white light. Bouncing like wheat chaff shaken on a screen, the twelve monkey zombies zinged and zanged and sang strange tunes. They bumped into each other, and into the gravestones, and stopped every few bounces to lick the walking stick.

As the three watched, a porcupine wandered into the circle. Two of the zombies bounced over and sniffed the animal. Sensing danger, the creature shot several of its quills into the nearest zombie, however, to no effect. One of the zombies opened up the porcupine's head and scooped out its brains.

"Ooh. Yucky!" Priscilla murmured.

Rashpewkin replied, "Look tasty to me."

Priscilla felt her stomach turn. "Maybe we should turn back. This is very scary. Jeri-Myah, what do you think?"

"They too bouncy," the frog replied. "Me can't get to stick."

"Rashpewkin have answer," the troll said. Reaching into his bag, he brought out the handful of candy he'd taken from the witch's house. "Give Zany Zombies coma candy. Maybe take away bounce?"

"And maybe it'll give them all a chance to suck out our brains," Priscilla said. "That candy might only work on living creatures. These zombies are likely to take the candy and take us too! How do we know they don't eat all living things?"

Rashpewkin pointed to the creatures. "Lookee. You see

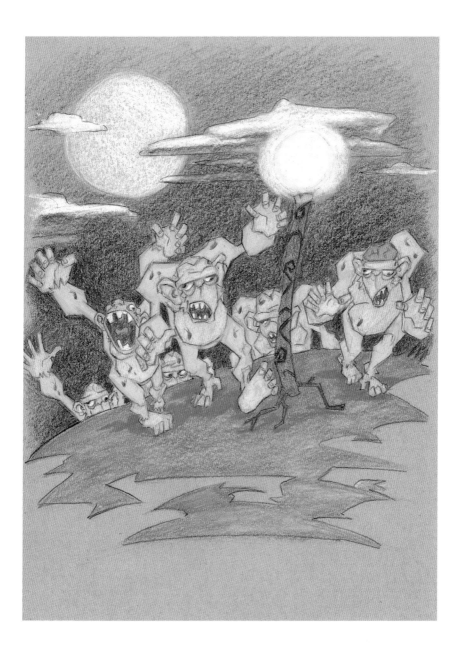

worms and flies all over them zombies?"

The princess squinted to see in the moonlight. Sure enough, the creatures all had a cloud of flying gnats and flies around them, and slimy-looking bugs and worms crawling in and out of their skin. "Ooh, double-yucky sloth soup. Why'd you have to point that out? As if I wasn't already going to have nightmares."

Jeri-Myah clapped. "See? Monkeys no eat bugs, so no eat frogs neither. Me give them candy."

Rashpewkin took the candy out of the bag and handed it to Jeri-Myah. The big frog took a deep breath and pushed through the bushes into the clearing. A greenish glowing zombie bounced up to her, took a sniff, and bounded away again.

Jeri-Myah held up a piece of candy to the next zombie that came her way. After sniffing the sweet, the zombie took a lick and bounced off. Whenever a monkey bounced up, it took a big lick. When the first candy was gone, Rashpewkin handed Jeri-Myah a second one, and then the third, until they'd gone through all the candy. With each lick, the creatures bounced away a bit slower. By the time the candy was gone, the dozen zombies no longer bounced. Instead, they strolled slowly, like leaves caught in a stream's whirlpool.

Jeri-Myah came back to the bushes, and Priscilla thrust the glass ball out at her. Grabbing it, she took it over to the stick where, reaching above her head, she placed the ball on the top of the stick. Even though the walking stick had no obvious flat surface, the ball balanced perfectly. Jeri-Myah hurried back to join Priscilla and Rashpewkin behind the bushes.

Glowing in the moonlight, the ball cast a blue iridescence that bounced off the zombies's eyes. Attracted to the light, they wandered up to the ball and licked it repeatedly. After several minutes, one by one, they fell to the ground and crawled into their graves. The dirt fell in on them and soon the only sounds Priscilla heard were the crickets and a distant hoot owl.

The three adventurers were just about to come out of hiding when the quiet shattered with the arrival of King Goethe and Prince Hector, charging into the clearing with their swords drawn.

"We're here, valiant knights of the Mystic Forest Kingdom, come to save the day!" Prince Hector shouted, slicing through some overhanging vines for emphasis.

Priscilla watched the king and prince rush around slashing at shadows. After tiring of that, they came up to the stick and pulled it up, knocking the ball to the ground. Holding the stick up high, King Goethe shouted, "Victory is ours!"

"Come on," Priscilla said. "Let's beat them back to camp."

"Jeri-Myah meet you soon," the frog said. "Get ball."

The princess and her troll made their way back to the tents, just settling in before hearing the voices of the men returning. When he reached the campsite, King Goethe called, "Wake up everyone. We've defeated the zombies."

Priscilla came out of her tent, stifling a yawn. When Prince Hector held the wonderful wooden weather wand up high for her to see she clapped in appreciation. She rushed forward and gave him a kiss.

"You're awesome, my handsome, strong, brave prince!"

He nodded. "Indeed I am!"

"How were the zombies?"

"No problem for brave knights like us." He pulled out his sword to demonstrate. "A swish and swash and we did them in. Quest accomplished in record time!"

King Goethe suggested they all get a few hours sleep and pack up in the morning. "If we push hard and have a little luck, we can get back to the castle by sunset." The two men headed into their tents.

Jeri-Myah came into the camp cuddling Fairy Freda's magic globe.

"What are you going to do with that?" Priscilla asked.

"Stare in, find kissing prince." She held it up to Priscilla's gaze, and for a moment she thought she saw Rashpewkin's likeness form before the sparkles turned back into meaningless swirls.

"So what do you think that means?" she asked.

"Be magic message. Rashpewkin help Jeri-Myah find prince, kiss, and turn back into real girl." She retreated to her tent, clutching the magic ball.

"I do hope she gets her wish," Priscilla said to Rashpewkin. "I'd hate to live my life as a warty old frog, wouldn't you?"

Rashpewkin stooped down and picked a caterpillar off the ground, popping it into his mouth. "Jeri-Myah no mind being frog. Never get hungry or angry."

"Oh? Why is that?"

Rashpewkin reached out his long tongue and snapped up a fly passing by. "'Cause eats whatever bugs her."

Chapter Ten: The Magical Kiss

King Goethe roused them shortly after dawn. Princess Priscilla dozed in the saddle as they rode, listening to her father and husband brag about their success, riding together ahead of her. Rashpewkin and Jeri-Myah gossiped on their donkey riding behind. Just after noon they stopped for a break near a small stream. Here they ate a lunch of freshly picked berries as they rested among the flowers.

Priscilla watched Rashpewkin and Jeri-Myah running barefoot through the blossoms. "Be careful you don't step on anything sharp," she called out.

Jeri-Myah held up a foot covered in flower blossoms. "See? Open toad shoes."

The two came and settled next to Priscilla, resting under a tree. She watched them snuggling together, Rashpewkin's arm around his cousin's shoulders.

"What are you thinking about?" the princess asked.

Rashpewkin sighed. "Remember when was real boy and Jeri-Myah real girl. We play all time. Good friends." He plucked a few dandelions and began twisting them into a chain. "Sure wish could be real boy again."

"What was it the obelisk said about that? Didn't it say that you'd already found that friend?" she asked. "What do you think that meant?"

Rashpewkin shrugged. "No know." He finished looping the chain upon itself, creating a necklace he placed around Jeri-Myah's neck. The frog gave it a twirl.

"You know frog's favorite flower?" she asked. "Crocus."

Priscilla stared from one to the other. "If Jeri-Myah is your cousin, is she of royal blood too?"

Rashpewkin nodded. "Yessiree. Distant cousin. She Uncle Remus daughter. He ruler of Kingdom of Briar Patch."

"So … doesn't that make her a royal princess?"

The two looked at each other, and Priscilla saw a distinct blush hit both their faces.

"That be true." Rashpewkin looked Jeri-Myah over as she lifted a hind leg and scratched behind her ear. "She be pretty girl then. Rashpewkin wonder what Jeri-Myah look like as woman."

"You two certainly like each other. Why not give her a kiss and see if you can break the spell?"

Rashpewkin's eyes brightened and he puckered up. Jeri-Myah looked at him shyly for a moment, and then grabbed him around the neck and covered his mouth with her thick bubbly lips. As they held the embrace they began changing, their limbs and trunks straightening out, their skins changing to a human pink. In a minute, instead of amphibian and reptile, two teenage humans held each other in loving embrace.

"Oh!" Priscilla exclaimed. "Look at you!"

Rashpewkin stood and jumped up and down. "Whoopee! Hurrah, hurray, hipp-hipp-horee! Look at me! I'm a boy! A real boy!"

"Indeed you both are human again!" Priscilla noted. "Hold on and we'll rustle up some clothes." She rummaged through her pack, bringing out a spare dress for Jeri-Myah and one of Hector's shirts for Rashpewkin. They dressed, the boy using a hanging vine he cut off as a belt.

King Goethe came up, looking at the pair in surprise. "What's happened here?"

"The spell is broken," Priscilla explained. "Rashpewkin and Jeri-Myah have turned back into humans."

The two kissed again, Jeri-Myah whispering, "I love you," and Rashpewkin smiling back tenderly.

"Well, well. Congratulations. Are you going to leave us like Boy Blue, or return to the castle?"

Rashpewkin bowed respectfully. "If it please Your Highness, I believe we'd like to return to my father's homeland. It's been almost ten years since I last saw him."

"Very well. You may take the donkey and your share of supplies. Also, here, as a wedding gift." The king pulled a handful of the leprechaun duggets from his coin purse and placed them into Rashpewkin's hand. "Should you wish to come visit, you will always be welcome in the Kingdom of the Mystic Forest."

Jeri-Myah curtsied and Rashpewkin bowed again. "We thank you, your Highness."

The remaining three mounted and continued their journey, reaching the castle just at sunset.

As they approached the moat they found a figure waiting for them, standing and blocking the drawbridge. Dressed in his brown cloak, Edgar the Evil Sorcerer leaned on the railing, a scowl across his face.

They rode up to him and the king called a halt. Dismounted, his arms crossed in front of his chest, he stood a few feet from the sorcerer. "What mean you to camp at our castle keep, you crusty curmudgeon? State your business or be off."

Edgar tapped his foot on the drawbridge's threshold. "Your Highness might consider treating his loyal subjects with more respect. Not that it bothers me much, but out of curiosity, what have I done to offend you?"

The king swept his arm towards the parched landscape, the Royal Terrace with its browned rose bushes and the Royal Garden with its wilted vegetables. "Your carelessness has caused our kingdom considerable inconvenience."

The sorcerer pulled his cloak tighter around his chest. "Yet, I believe you've now recovered my wonderful wooden weather wand. You vanquished the zombies?"

Prince Hector alighted from his steed and swaggered up to the sorcerer. "Indeed! We worthy warriors verily vanquished the fiendish foes. With abounding aptitudes, we ablated the abysmal abhorrent abnormals, abolishing the abusive aborigines, absconding with the aberrant aberrancy, abjuring their objections."

Edgar grunted. "Oh, so very impressive. Scared off a handful of dead monkeys, and I suppose you think you're the dragon's breath now?"

Prince Hector pulled out his sword and raised it menacingly. "We are brave knights of the Mystic Forest and know well how to deal with miscreants."

Edgar gave his magic wand a flick and Hector's sword clunked to the ground. "A lead sword might slow down your meaningless threats."

While the men stood glaring at each other, Priscilla climbed off her steed and took the wonderful wooden weather wand off the king's saddle. Handing it over to the sorcerer, she said, "We really need you to bring rain."

After a few more grumbles, the sorcerer raised his stick to the skies, waving it around as he mumbled a tongue-twisting spell. He pounded the staff on the ground thrice. In the distance, the roar of thunder echoed back. Within minutes, thick gray clouds covered the sky.

The three castle staff came out, drawn by the commotion. "Blackburn," the king called to the blacksmith, "take the horses into the stable. The rest of you, get inside. Looks like it's going to be a storm!"

He turned to Edgar. "We magnanimously accept your pleas for mercy. As you're offering appropriate restitution for the harm

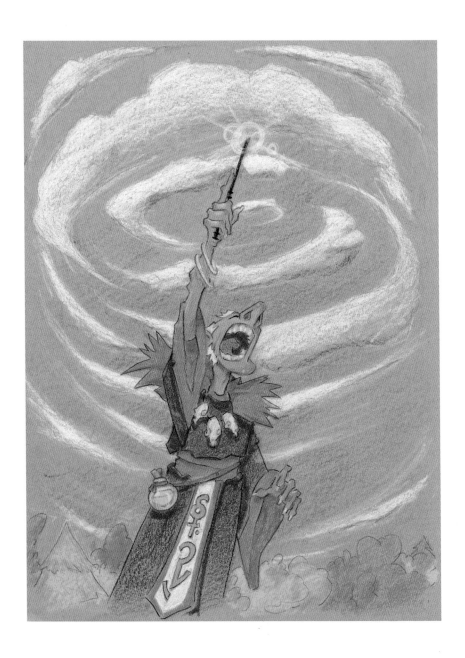

you've brought to our kingdom, I grant you pardon for this offense."
Shaking his finger at the sorcerer he added, "But be forewarned, I
may not be so lenient next time."

Edgar sneered. "Oh how very generous of you, Your Highness.
Now, I have my own business to attend to." Pointedly ignoring them
as he walked past, he trudged down the path towards the village as
the first drops of rain began to fall.

Later that evening, Priscilla and Hector watched the
thunderstorm from the window of their castle bedroom. The water
from the moat, overfilled by the continuing rains, tumbled out of the
bloated creek and down through the meadow.

"This downpour dampens the dreadful drought," Hector
noted.

"Yes, it's good to be home and safe. I hope we can stay that
way for awhile. You and Daddy seem to want to jump into adventure
at the slightest whim."

He pulled her into a tight hug and kissed her on the forehead.
"That's what valiant knights do, my princess. Besides, no one can
predict the future … unless he has a magic globe."

"Oh!" Princess pushed away and went to her bag. Rummaging
through, she pulled out the magic ball she'd gotten back from Jeri-
Myah. She brought it back to the windowsill, and together she and

Hector gazed into it. As the storm raged, flecks of color and shapes coalesced in the globe. Slowly it formed into the shape of a big wolf.

"Look!" Priscilla shouted. "Werewolves!"

"Where wolves?" Hector asked standing to look out the window.

"Oh, never mind, my brave knight. I'm sure we'll see them soon enough."

The End

About the Author

Diagnosed with polio at age fourteen, Philip's mother, Beatrice, took up typing to keep her fingers nimble. She became a professional writer, on staff with the WWII US Army "Stars and Stripes," awarded a PhD in English literature, and publishing thirty books and over a thousand stories and articles. Franklyn Levin, Philip's father, took up poetry after retiring at age 65, scribing over 200 poems by age 90. With these role models, Philip took up writing at a young age, publishing a small book as a child, editing his college newspaper, and paying his medical school tuition from articles he sold.

"I love telling stories," Philip said. "I write in all genres, beginning with my murder mystery *Inheritance*, I've tried my hand at contemporary romance, children's photo books, bible stories, and fiction and nonfiction anthologies. Some of my favorite tales are stories based on the cases I see in my job as an emergency room physician."

Traveling to far corners of the world, Philip has found inspiration from lepers in India, impoverished orphans in rural Kenya, water buffalo farmers in China, and nature reserves in the Galapagos Islands. His poetry has won statewide contests in several regions, and his short stories and articles have appeared in over two-dozen magazines.

"Children fantasy remains one of my favorite genres," he reported. "This book was inspired by my insatiable childhood reading, with references from nursery rhymes, children's books, and even cartoons. It's full of fun and puns and will bring a smile to readers of all ages."

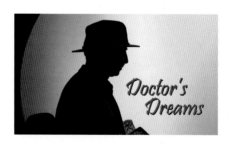

Contact Dr. Levin at writerpllevin@gmail.com
Peruse his books at www.Doctors-Dreams.com